Conducting With **Dementia** In The family

"A unique and great read for those having daily to confront dementia in the family. It is a positive and uplifting approach. A must buy for all with this dilemma."

Professor Sir Cary L. Cooper CBE
Distinguished Professor of Organizational Psychology
and Health, Lancaster University

"In this easy to read and understand book, psychoanalyst Trevor Mumby offers hope of well-being to the many family care givers who are supporting a loved one suffering with dementia. Trevor has found a route out of the despair and frustration so often experienced by dedicated family members. Anyone who wants help in caring for this condition will find this excellent work a revelation."

Joyce Hunt, Geratologist. RN Specialist Nurse
Practitioner for Older People, New South Wales, Australia

'This book is a timely and essential reading for caregivers of people with dementia, as a way of understanding that the medical approach is not the only solution.'

Professor Philip Poi Jun Hua. Senior Consultant in
Geriatric Medicine at The University of Malaya,
Kuala Lumpur

Conducting Well-Being With **Dementia** In The family

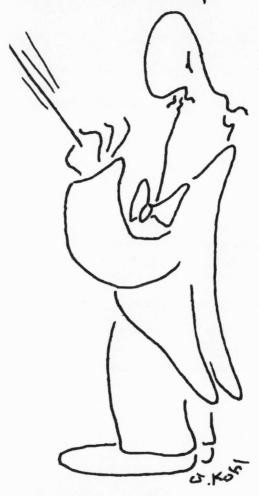

Trevor Mumby

authorHOUSE®

AuthorHouse™ UK
1663 Liberty Drive
Bloomington, IN 47403 USA
www.authorhouse.co.uk
Phone: 0800.197.4150

Published by AuthorHouse 02/23/2015

ISBN: 978-1-5049-3806-8 (sc)
ISBN: 978-1-5049-3807-5 (hc)
ISBN: 978-1-5049-3809-9 (e)

Print information available on the last page.

Any people depicted in stock imagery provided by Thinkstock are models, and such images are being used for illustrative purposes only.
Certain stock imagery © Thinkstock.

Contents

Preface

After completing an apprenticeship as a motor engineer, at the age of 20, Trevor's life took on a complete change. He was drafted into the Royal Army Medical Corp where he trained as a mental nurse before working in mental health wards in both the UK and Singapore.

On returning from Singapore he started working and living in mental aftercare homes before attending Glasgow University where he graduated in Social Study and Edinburgh University in Psychiatric Social Work.

Trevor undertook a Jungian training analysis at the Davidson Clinic in Edinburgh and moved to London to work in the Mental Health Social Services. During this period he undertook training analysis at the Group Analytic Practice (London).

He has worked in various parts of the world

as a consultant in organisational behaviour for a number of multinational companies during which time he graduated with an M.SC in Organisation Development.

For the past 12 years he has been co-director of a company providing care services to the elderly. The company has around 90 staff who attend specialist dementia courses specifically designed and conducted by Trevor. He is also conducting 'Training The Trainer' courses in Australia with plans to run similar courses in the USA.

He is a Senior Associate Member of The Royal Society of Medicine, Associate Member of the American Group Psychotherapy Association and also a Member of the British Association of Social Workers.

His publications include; *The Large Group in Industry. In The Large Group, the Dementia and You Action Pack* and *Coaching for Carers - A fresh look at dementia care.*

The Courses

It has become plain that as a result of Trevor's training courses, staff and family members gain a deeper understanding from each other when the principle learning comes through the *experiential* process of group membership.

Each member has a unique personality and an absolutely unique relationship with their cared-for person. There are NO off-the-shelf solutions. A group of up to eight people meet for one hour sessions on a weekly or twice-weekly basis. Each member will have studied Trevor's manual; *Coaching for Carers - A Fresh Look at Dementia Care*, which they are given before the course starts and are expected to use throughout the six sessions of the course.

The interpersonal dynamics within the group evoke patterns of behaviour which individuals begin to recognise as 'hand-grenades' which cause negative reactions within the group. After six hours of group conversation, the members have fine-tuned themselves and find their interpersonal relations, both in and out of the group, much more enjoyable and less 'explosive' in the presence of their cared-for person.

These courses have proven to transform not only the home environment but the family and wider networks such as neighbours and visiting professionals.

For the past 10 years, Trevor has frequently visited relatives and witnessed the intense difficulties of families experiencing a loved one undergoing the dreadful process of dementia.

He is profoundly aware of the difficult family circumstances where relatives have absolutely NO IDEA how they can cope except by doing the best they can...*it hurts*!

There is NO DOUBT in his mind that 99.99% of them are, with all the love in world, exacerbating their problems WITHOUT KNOWING. They cannot do anything except *be themselves* and do the best they can.

This is NOT a Do-It-Yourself handbook it is a Be-It-Yourself workbook. By all means read it a few times, it is not rocket science and will not take up too much of your precious time.

If you really want to live successfully with someone experiencing the behaviour caused by dementia, the ESSENTIAL skill will be for you to identify YOURSELF with the confusion that the person experiences and their increasing inability to live in YOUR world.

In his opinion there is an almost worldwide and false belief that LOSS OF MEMORY is the overwhelming problem associated with dementia.

It is commonly believed that if we can somehow 'jog' their memory with some extremely clever memory jogging devices, we will be contributing immensely to their well-being.

WRONG!

If we could identify with a mental state of ever increasing CONFUSION and be confused *ourselves*, it would all begin to make sense!

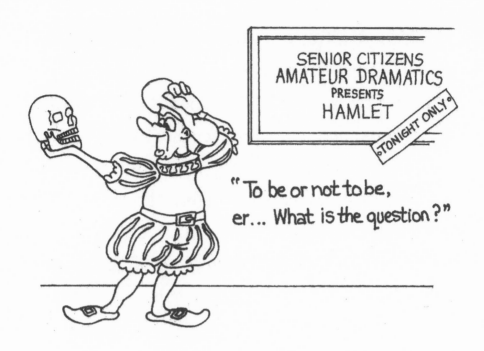

"To be or not to be, er... What is the question?"

"Of course I forget things! *You would if you got as confused as I do!*"

"Of course I get angry when people assume I AM NOT CONFUSED! *You would!*"

"Of course I am not going to trust you to help with my confusion, when you think all that is wrong with me is that I forget things and treat me like an idiot!"

"I don't want my memory jogging, thank you very much."

"I am still here behind my confusion, not some absent-minded person, needing sympathetic memory jogging!"

"The ordinary arts we practice every day at home are of more importance to the soul than their simplicity might suggest."

Thomas Moore

Introduction

It came as a huge surprise when after six months of scanning the internet for sites relating to dementia and Alzheimer's Disease, all I found was thousands of words advising us what to DO and how to do all types of things FOR the person with the problem. There was an over whelming, underlying assumption that THEY NEEDED IT.

As if there were a CURE and they would all get better!

I thought, what if we approached it from the opposite direction?

What can we learn?

We need them!

The set of assumptions this creates calls for a very different approach and mental attitude.

This maybe greeted warmly by some and with anger by others. The challenge it presents is to do with ONE basic assumption, which needs to be established if pleasure and well-being are to be the predominant emotions for the future...

I am the person who needs to do ALL of the changing . . . **if I want to!**

My loved one CANNOT.

Welcome to DEMENTIA WORLD

GOLDEN RULE ONE

Please make every effort to REFRAIN from using common sense, remember; YOU are the one who CAN change. The person for whom you care; has NO CHOICE. Their future contentedness can be devastated by well-meaning, common sense, unaware interactions which re-stimulate trauma and negative feelings.

GOLDEN RULE TWO

You are not TREATING A PATIENT and the term should be totally divorced from your mind. We do not have patients with dementia, we have behaviour changes, which we are challenged to understand and communicate with.

GOLDEN RULE THREE

We HAVE to focus on the NOW and not wait for a 'miracle' cure in the future.

"Despite all efforts to the contrary, as the second decade of the 21st century dawns, biomedical efforts to delay, prevent, or cure dementia are showing no significant success."

Professor Stephen Post. Stony Brook University. NY

You will be developing a whole new set of life skills, that will greatly enhance your own quality of life and profoundly influence the course that the dementia will take.

Please make thorough notes because I guarantee that you WILL see significant changes and it is vital for everyone to benefit from these observations. YOU are learning and your main teacher will be the person for whom you care, who will give you a roller coaster ride! The people who may be supporting you must learn from YOU, but remember...

"When someone whom
I have helped,
or in whom I have placed
great hopes,
mistreats me in extremely
hurtful ways,
I regard him still as my
precious teacher."

The Dalai Lama

We simply have not been taught how to conduct our lives!

What did our school teach us about how to become a millionaire? Or, become a mental and physical role model for our spouse and the children we might have as we grew older? Or, see the vast universe of potential, life-enriching opportunities there are on planet Earth?

What did it teach about the most vital skill from which any human being would gain a LIFELONG means to acquire serenity and a sharp intelligent mind?

Did ANY of us leave our educational days, fully able to use mind-relaxing skills, which give us competence and tranquility when faced with what life was going to throw at us?

No!

14

Now! Those of us who are living our lives in relationships where everyday can be challenging and filled with emotional hand grenades, MUST be able to call upon some skills which help us to transcend these circumstances with EASE!

Having never learned them before, try learning them NOW.

1. Find a nice quiet space which is free of distractions. It takes careful thought but when you inspect the space, you will be surprised how many distractions there are which you may never have considered.

2. Find a comfortable upright chair, sit on it, take off your shoes and place your hands comfortably on your lap. Lower your eyes so that they are not 'working' and also not about to lull you into sleep.

3. Busy your mind by recalling very happy memories from ANY period in your life. Just work on that one task until you can say to yourself, 'that's it for now'.

The importance of this exercise cannot be over emphasised.

What you will be doing, is locating, from your lifetime, happy feelings about which you will instantly be able to describe minute details AND LAUGH SPONTANEOUSLY!

It will take you sometime, but I guarantee it will happen. You should be able to regenerate laughing moments from at least three different time periods.

Please write down key words for EACH moment.

THEY ARE UNIQUE TO YOU!

Only YOU know how funny the events were.

4. Keeping that experience flowing in your mind, begin attending to your breathing. You are feeling happy, even smiling to yourself, and noticing your breathing. Don't care about your breathing, just let it go on without you interfering with it! It is unique to you!

5. The anchor which is holding you calmly in the

bouncing sea of distracting thoughts, will be made of YOUR OWN LAUGHTER EXPERIENCES. Keep them and use them at any moment when you feel threatened by negativity.

You will be sitting relaxed with your feet firmly resting on the floor, your hands sitting comfortably on your lap, your breathing flowing effortless with you and your happy memories bobbing around in the tidal swell of the many distracting thoughts flowing in and out of your mind.

EASY isn't it? No tricks, no gimmicks, just intelligent you spending time for yourself. Ten minutes, at least twice a day and very soon you will be telling everyone to do it!

I guarantee that you will acquire a routine specifically unique for YOU which ALWAYS results in you transcending the stresses and worries which maybe oppressing you. You learn to become an excellent life manager!

Lots of different methods which can be incorporated into this process are listed in the appendix, at the end of this book.

The inadvertent use of 'HAND GRENADES!'

Over the years, with many thousands of hours working with interpersonal complexities, I have concluded that there are twelve characteristics in our behavior which are completely natural. Like fish in water, these twelve make up the element in which we all 'swim'.

In everyday relationships any one, or combinations, of these 'natural' elements can be the cause of disharmony and argument but are relatively harmless.

Any one of these used in the presence of someone experiencing the massive confusion caused through a brain disease, CAN cause an *EXPLOSION*.

Opinionating
Interrupting
Provoking
Contradicting
Expecting gratitude
Talking Loudly
Undermining
Pessimism
Ignoring
Need to control
Questioning
Irritating

We will be demonstrating this later, the critical reality which I dearly hope will reveal itself through your wisdom is that we, in our everyday natural element, doing what comes naturally to us, are throwing 'hand grenades' into the confused world of our cared-for person by using any one of them without sensitive awareness.

It is these explosions which through their use, cause the effects in behaviour which seems so incredibly difficult to live with and which generate the tension and stress in our lives.

We have to be calm and composed with the knowledge, through our awareness, of their potential damage.

WE carry the hand grenades!!!

The FRESH look

When dementia begins to affect people,
CONFUSION takes over. Remember, this is a
Be-It-Yourself workbook.

The survey here is intended for you to take
a snapshot of yourself before you complete the
guiding exercises.

ON A SCALE OF 1-10 HOW FREQUENTLY DO I . . .

	1	2	3	4	5	6	7	8	9	10
Opinionate:	☐	☐	☐	☐	☐	☐	☐	☐	☐	☐
Interrupt:	☐	☐	☐	☐	☐	☐	☐	☐	☐	☐
Provoke:	☐	☐	☐	☐	☐	☐	☐	☐	☐	☐
Contradict:	☐	☐	☐	☐	☐	☐	☐	☐	☐	☐
Expect Gratitude:	☐	☐	☐	☐	☐	☐	☐	☐	☐	☐
Talk Loudly:	☐	☐	☐	☐	☐	☐	☐	☐	☐	☐
Undermine:	☐	☐	☐	☐	☐	☐	☐	☐	☐	☐
Act Pessimistic:	☐	☐	☐	☐	☐	☐	☐	☐	☐	☐
Ignore:	☐	☐	☐	☐	☐	☐	☐	☐	☐	☐
Control:	☐	☐	☐	☐	☐	☐	☐	☐	☐	☐
Ask Questions:	☐	☐	☐	☐	☐	☐	☐	☐	☐	☐
Irritate:	☐	☐	☐	☐	☐	☐	☐	☐	☐	☐

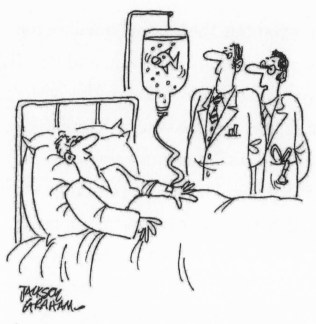

"WE FIND IT CALMS THE PATIENT."

ACQUIRING CALM

This is the number one PRIORITY lesson for which you MUST find time EVERY DAY for 5 to 15 minutes. *NO EXCUSES!!!*

From our earlier exercise, you will have reminded yourself about your laughter memories and instantly experienced the well-being they bring to you.

When you learn a calming technique, your calmness begins to have a profound effect, not only on you but the person you care for.

They will 'catch' your calm and BELIEVE ME, you will see and feel serenity, perhaps never experienced by you or your cared-for person BEFORE dementia started!

It will be very helpful if you find a visual image that refreshes your sense of peace, put it where you will see it, and place some speakers around so that you can occasionally play music which you both enjoy.

One other INEVITABLE result from these calming sessions is that clear thoughts will be released effortlessly *(to your surprise at first)*, and give YOU more understanding about the best things you can do.

The ONLY goal is to establish and retain a sense of well-being for YOURSELF, because from there, you radiate *your* sense of calm confidence!

When you have become skilled in calming your own feelings and seen the peaceful

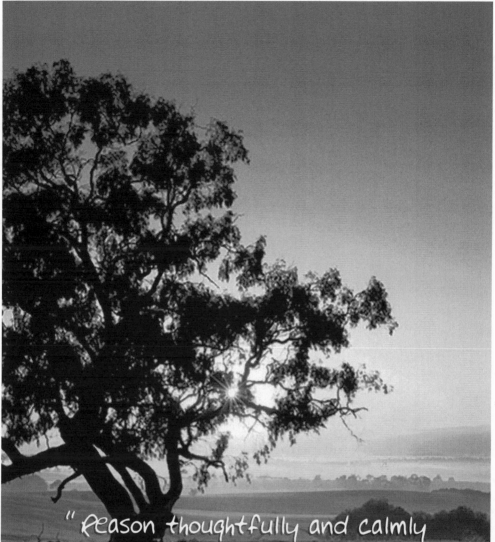

" Reason thoughtfully and calmly
and choose from these answers which
one seems the best way to conduct
your life and if you do this not
only your own life but the lives of
others around you will become
better and better."

Robert M Pirsig.
Foreword in Coffee with Plato by Donald R Moor

results, you have *only just started!*

However good you become at calming and establishing a peaceful atmosphere, there are many potential traps into which you can fall! This next part of the exercises, starts AFTER you have practiced enough to have a glimpse of a peaceful state of mind and look forward to the time when you can give yourself another calming session.

Even in our normal lives, we constantly conduct ourselves in a manner which creates discordant responses and disharmony by using mannerisms which we have grown up with and taken as our natural behaviour!

Regardless of how blissfully happy you are and completely free of dementia, the above habits, beliefs and mannerisms lurk in the NORMAL relating of everyday life.

Test yourself! Imagine YOU have a fragile grasp of the world around you and feel you are on the fringes of sanity.

What effect would happen if only ONE

of these habits, beliefs and mannerisms is discordant, never mind the remaining eleven?

Being confused can become the status quo. *Everything confuses you.*

Opinionating

It is so natural for us to treasure our opinions and protect them to extraordinary lengths, even in the face of facts which contradict them!

Spend one whole day expressing an opinion with people you meet during the day. It will be incredibly revealing, especially if the opinions you voice are ones you genuinely hold!

At the end of the day, please list how many nice people you encountered and also how many questionable people.

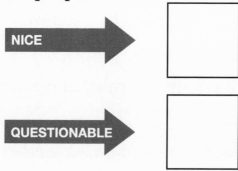

If you learn anything it will again be a shock.

"Am I so opinionated?"

Formulating ANY opinion *(right or wrong)* is INCREDIBLY important for a person doubting their sanity. To have it challenged, will probably feel devastating.

In the presence of a person experiencing dementia, keep your opinions to yourself.

YOUR OPINIONATING EXERCISE

This is the type of mannerism, which OTHER people demonstrate, certainly NOT you!

Just to prove it. Please start a conversation with people you know about sex, religion or politics.

After you have been talking for about 10 minutes and are thoroughly engaged, stay silent for while and listen to the others.

Your observations will tell you something about whether or not YOU opinionate with people who have dementia and the effect it might be having on their feelings.

Having an opinion AT ALL when confusion reigns is like having an anchor to hold you safely.

Please AGREE with your cared-for person, whatever their opinion. Their well-being is your primary objective. YOUR opinion can be expressed elsewhere! Write notes for yourself here and on the next page.

What have I observed about opinions?

_____

_____

_____

_____

_____

_____

_____

Interrupting

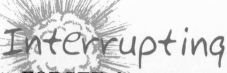

I want you to **FORGET** the person you care for and go shopping! Spend two hours doing your normal thing! You are calm, peaceful and smiling to yourself. Now . . . LISTEN!

Try to hear how many times you interrupt, how many times others interrupt you and how many times you hear other people interrupting each other. I wager that you will be shocked.

Please write down on this page the number of times interruption was evident in your normal healthy life on this shopping trip.

That number represents constant blocking of thought processes!

Can you imagine how it FEELS for your cared-for person, even if the number was halved? To counteract these thought blocking habits which are perfectly normal;

Allow your cared-for person to finish their sentences and let them lead from the moment you observe their effort to converse with you.

Doing this is a high skill and incredibly satisfying when it becomes effortless. EVERYONE with whom you converse, especially the person with dementia, can notice the evidence of its effectiveness.

We frequently hear from relatives that they are being told things from the past which they had never heard before!

<u>YOUR INTERRUPTING EXERCISE</u>

This exercise is FUN. Don't let anyone tell you, YOU DON'T interrupt!

All you need to do is go about your daily activities and observe OTHER people.

When you have done it for long enough, you will have no doubt about how common it is.

For your next challenge, restrain yourself from interrupting in ANY conversation and note the difference. A good example to test yourself with, is when your cared-for person keeps repeating themselves. It is SO tempting to interrupt! Don't forget you are with a very confused person, they need to remove their confusion in WHATEVER they do.

Observe their reaction to you. They might look quite surprised when you don't interrupt and start to chat to you. Be patient and let them lead the way.

Try to write notes for yourself below.
Do I interrupt often? What happens if I stop?

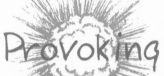

Provoking

This is not only a feature which stems from our behaviour, it often stems from the immediate ENVIRONMENT and can be totally invisible to people NOT experiencing dementia.

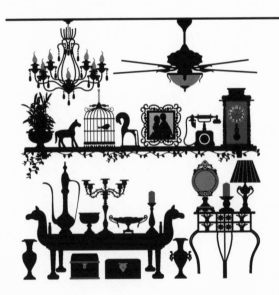

Which one of these do you think would provoke YOU?

The learning for this exercise calls for YOU to become a detective! Spend a week simply observing your cared-for person's reactions.

Not only reactions to you or visitors but MORE IMPORTANTLY, the rooms they go in and out of. The objects, colours, the light and shade, the pictures, photographs, the radio when it is on, the TV and the temperature.

Please SEE their environment and detect their reactions to it.

This exercise will highlight the extent to which CERTAIN features cause a smile and a relaxing response and others, a negative, tense, avoiding response.

It can become possible to re–assemble living areas and transform them into more relaxing and less provocative places.

<u>YOUR PROVOKING EXERCISE</u>

One of the strange things about being provoked is that the cause cannot be identified without clever detective work.

It need not be caused by personal behaviour but by something in the surroundings, which only affects YOU.

When you are reacting to a provocation, your friends might even say, "What is upsetting you?"

Try to make notes about things, which provoke you. It may be other people or situations, sights, sounds, tastes, smells, dark/light, memories, objects, colours, comments. The list might be surprising!

NOW. When you are with the person who is experiencing dementia, become a detective! You know what provokes YOU; begin to observe what might be provoking the cared-for person and be surprised, sometimes a room is full of hidden 'land mines'. E.g. a photograph which restimulates bad feelings about the place, time, circumstances or people at the moment it was taken.

Try to write notes for yourself opposite.

What provokes me? And the person I care for?

Contradiction

My wife and I are stopped by a passing motorist who asks us the way to a local farm.

"Ah that's easy," I say, and start to give the person directions.

My wife chips in and says "Oh no dear, it is the second left, not the first"

I collect my thoughts, as any rational man would and say, "Oh yes dear, you are right".

I then continue and my wife chips in again and says "No dear, it is AFTER The Crown, not before". This time I knew I was right!

"No darling, it IS before the Crown"

The motorist is looking confused.

I insisted that it is before The Crown and he should watch out for the school on his left around 100 meters before the farm gate.

"Oh no dear, that would be far too late. He would drive straight past," etc, etc.

This normal contradictory exchange would

leave us both saying something like;

'We must have really confused the poor man."

This mild, 'normal' interaction, when in the company of someone who may be confused already, will be like another hand grenade.

Their confusion intensifies and they will probably get very angry and tell you to *'Get out!'*

Contradiction is NORMAL. Our use of it is normal. In dementia world, it is a lethal weapon!

YOUR CONTRADICTION EXERCISE

This raises its head and causes NO stir because it seems to be an everyday common habit. We don't even register it until, for example, we are with friends and a stranger asks for directions to the nearest supermarket. You describe your route and your friends all tell the stranger a very different, more confusing route! How do YOU feel?

In order to reveal its predominant power in everyday conversation you will have to place yourself in a group, listen to a chat show, or whatever is popular.

Simply count the number of contradictions. It requires some disciplined listening and after a time you will become tuned into the habit.

It is one of those styles of conversing, of which you will become very aware when you do it to others!

Please note that because it is SUBTLE, a person with a clear, unconfused mind might hear it and let it go.

With someone experiencing dementia, who is struggling to retain a sense of intelligent awareness, it is a hand grenade!

Try catching yourself in various conversations and see if you can hear yourself contradicting the person with whom you are in conversation.

I heard myself contradicting .... times. I have reduced the frequency and the effects are:

..

..

What have I learned today?

_____

_____

_____

_____

_____

_____

_____

_____

_____

_____

_____

_____

Expecting gratitude

"Gratitude is a duty, which ought to be paid, but which none have a right to expect."

Jean-Jacques Rousseau

Common sense tells us that we would normally express gratitude to anyone who does something for us for which we are sincerely grateful.

We commonly expect to give or receive it. We grow up with it ingrained in our normal life. When it isn't given, we normally experience resentment, however trivial it might seem. That is NORMAL.

If we examine our expectations, we might find that we EXPECT gratitude for the 'sacrifices' we are making, forgetting that the concept of gratitude no longer exists in the confused mind of someone with dementia.

Remember, it is I who must change and it is I who should be grateful to them.

This state of mind will gradually emerge from the insights you are gaining and the behaviour changes which are taking place.

You can expect tons of gratitude from whomever you like, EXCEPT the cared-for person. You will have to learn to accept that because it is no longer a part of their everyday repertoire *and they are fantastic teachers!*

YOUR GRATITUDE EXERCISE

No-one who experiences the non-recognition they receive from their life-long partner, brother, sister, dad or mum who is experiencing dementia, will ever get over the hurt it first caused. The recovery and adjustment process from this upsetting interaction may take a very long time.

When the NEW person emerges from the perceptions that had been ingrained over a lifetime, it will give the opportunity to make a revolutionary insight!

This is a NEW person with a brain disease.

Spouse, brother, sister, dad, mum, what are they teaching me? What am I learning?

Am I thanking him/her for opening my eyes to fresh life experiences?

It is fine to be grateful for the life-long gifts you may have received but the gifts you COULD be receiving might even outweigh those from the past! Try to make a note for yourself below. Do I expect gratitude? What if it's not there?

Talking loudly

This is another one of those mannerisms which is common and will only cause offence when it is too loud for anyone around to have a normal conversation. *"I can't hear myself think!"*

The exercise is meant for you to spend time listening to YOURSELF in normal every day conversations.

YOUR TALKING LOUDLY EXERCISE

The exercise is meant for you to spend time listening to YOURSELF in normal everyday conversations.

There is an audible level of conversation between people, which demonstrates three golden qualities. People are LISTENING, HEARING (understanding) and RESPONDING in a way which harmonises the conversation and not creating a discordant 'noise'. In other words, they are NOT talking to themselves but believing they are talking to someone who is listening!

Give yourself one week with this one because it can become fun and once you have acquired the knack, you will enjoy observing how talking loudly is totally unacceptable to a person experiencing dementia. The opposite needs to happen. Calm, clear, subdued, harmonised conversation produces well-being.

Try to make a note for yourself below. What have I learned this week about volume?

_____

_____

_____

_____

_____

_____

_____

DISCOVERING DEMENTIA WORLD

The learning being acquired on this path should be reaching a level where the whole world perspective from *common sense* to *dementia sense* is coming into focus.

You are finding yourself being different.

You now know that giving attention in dementia world is very different. It is NOT about not ignoring *(common sense),* it is about your calm being transferred and the consequences this causes.

You are smiling more frequently, your voice level has dropped, and you physically touch your cared-for person more frequently. You have begun enjoying living in the dementia world, AS WELL AS your common sense world.

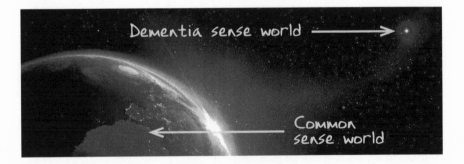

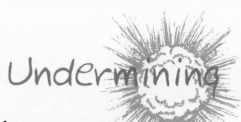

Undermining

Undermining competences

There is a universal recognition of ageism and anyone who APPEARS to be over a certain age will categorically confirm its prevalence by the subtle undermining of his or her sense of competence. Being undermined at any age is demoralising.

Your cared-for person is hypersensitive to being undermined and if this has been an insidious, imperceptible element in normal relations, it dramatically erupts into volcanic proportions.

The need to acknowledge INTELLIGENCE becomes paramount. You may be seeing increasing faltering and confusion but feelings of intelligence must not be undermined.

Diminishing comprehension will certainly be causing them HUGE frustration, which may well be expressed through anger.

The need to express your feelings of pride in their verbal expression and comprehension becomes paramount.

TRY BEING AN UNDERMINED PERSON YOURSELF . . . ?

YOUR UNDERMINING EXERCISE

The effects of being "put-down" or undermining our self-confidence is frequently demonstrated to us as children.

We are growing up and acquiring fresh knowledge and status from our peers. It is important to us that these successes from child to adult are preserved. Our well-being depends on a sense of self-confidence.

This exercise is intended for you to recall the schoolmates and teachers who supported and respected you in your early years.

As dementia begins to erode self-confidence and feelings of well-being for your cared-for person, it is CRUEL to put-down or undermine someone who is struggling with confusion about who they are.

Name as many of your favourite people and rate them with a score of 1-10 for their reinforcement of your well-being and self-confidence. The ones with high scores will make excellent role models.

Who are my favourite people? How do they rate?

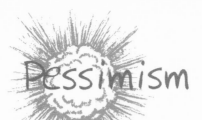Pessimism

There is overwhelming evidence that a child's esteem is severely influenced by the attitude and beliefs expressed by their teachers. The whole of a child's future can be limited by the pessimism of their teachers.

Unfortunately, pessimism is very common and widely expressed. It is perfectly understandable for carers to express it.

The question for us is; How much is it a part of our NORMAL daily interactions and can we rein it in?

If you have progressed this far, my bet is that you have found yourself getting calmer, less like the 'normal' person you were before dementia appeared and probably feeling pleased with the changes which have taken place.

This exercise will confound you and your close friends! Negativity is EVERYWHERE. The fun available to you is to consciously note it and log the sheer quantity, which surrounds you.

Make notes for a week – *places, BBC, (newsprint), friends, shopkeepers, etc.*

Shopkeeper held at knifepoint

Tsunami kills thousands

Hosepipe ban on the way

Banks in meltdown

When you review your notes PLEASE look INSIDE yourself and describe the feelings you are experiencing. Isn't it shocking, the extent to which nothing YOU have said or done could have avoided what has been your experience over the week? Do you want to spend the rest of your life as a victim of pessimism?

The way to totally neutralize it in your everyday relations with the person experiencing the helplessness dementia can induce is to: *CONSTANTLY COUNTERACT PESSIMISM!*

YOUR PESSIMISM EXERCISE

This is an epidemic! Pessimism radiates negative vibrations from every type of media. It is the most popular mannerism and easily the best way to join in a conversation. e.g. "The weather is awful today isn't it?"

The fact that pessimism is contagious, requires care-givers with those experiencing dementia, to positively COUNTERACT and defend their cared-for person from its overwhelming impact.

Everyone will need to do it according to his or her personal circumstances but to take it on, first complete the following exercise.

Go shopping! Hear it, see it and record the number of occurrences!

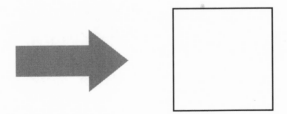

How am I affected by the level of pessimism?

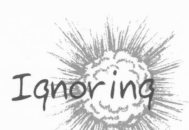

Ignoring

In everyday relations, ignoring is so prevalent that the phrase *"Yes dear,"* can be a flippant, benignly accepted phrase meaning s/he is not really interested in what I have said, done or about to do.

Again, if we look at dementia world, we will instantly observe that ignoring takes on a powerfully more explosive significance.

The NEED to know is vital, for enforcing a sense of sanity. What were almost amusing throwaway phrases like *"Yes dear,"* are heard as *"YES DEAR, WHAT!!!!"*

Dementia magnifies the need for attention a hundredfold!

Try being the ignored person yourself.

YOUR IGNORING EXERCISE

The most vivid demonstration of being ignored will be one of those hurtful memories still being stored in YOUR memory bank. Observing it in the home of someone experiencing dementia will hurt anyone who is also sensitive towards being ignored.

"How CAN they do that?"

Of course it is quite harmless most of the time and when it is pointed out, there is an immediate apology from the ignorer.

Again I have to say, if YOU are sensitive to it, what about the person struggling to know; who, what or where is anything? Being ignored is what they DO NOT want.

The exercise here is for you to go into your normal living pattern for long enough to notice how much ignoring is going on around you and OF you! If you are ignoring people, it may well be something you do to others without being aware.

Try to write a note for yourself below.
Am I often ignored? Do I ignore others?

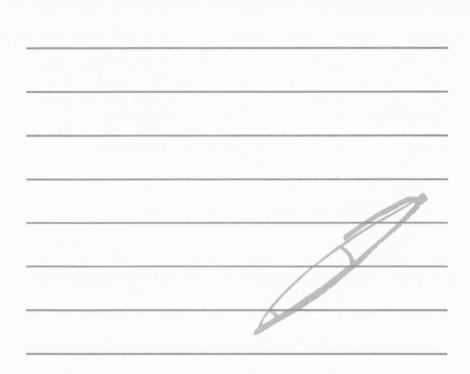

Controlling

In the normal world we use the phrase 'henpecked' to describe control being applied by a wife to a husband. The term; male chauvinist pig, usually describes a husband doing the same thing, himself.

Unfortunately, our need for control equates to our fear of outright chaos and EVERY situation can become potentially uncontrollable. People with a heightened fear of losing control are unkindly described as 'control freaks'.

It is easy to imagine how such a person will respond to the frequently random 'out of control' behaviour of their cared-for person when their behaviour becomes highly erratic.

If the need to control was part of their pre-dementia relationship, the partner with this need will most definitely find it will become 'nightmare-ish' for them.

To round off this section, I want to suggest that the need for control arises not only from fear of chaos and disorder but a lack of ideas about how to cope when faced with the fear.

New ideas might not come from within the 'box' of normal common sense thinking but there is an excellent chance that ideas WILL emerge from the calming sessions you are doing.

The final exercise therefore. is to take your thinking about your fear of losing control into your calming session, and as you achieve that state of calm, solutions will 'float' into your intelligence which make it crystal clear how YOU will be discarding your need to control.

I hope that these exercises have helped you to see your common sense self and the effects these normal everyday patterns can have on behaviour when you are in the presence of someone experiencing a brain disease.

In the next section, we say it is often the well-intentioned inappropriate actions of the caregivers which might well be causing desperate feelings. Being in dementia world and learning how to conduct interpersonal and environmental 'music', will have a powerful effect on the well-being of everyone, especially you, because YOU can be the fount of calm well-being.

<u>YOUR CONTROLLING EXERCISE</u>
We all have a tendency to control others,

especially if we think we know best. The need to control, or be controlled, is not unusual.

When caring, we frequently take on a mannerism of protecting our cared-for person and in the case of young children or people with patterns of behaviour which may be a danger to themselves or others, that is an appropriate action.

The difference when caring for someone experiencing dementia, especially in the early phases, is that controlling feels to them like you are ASSUMING they have become dependent and incapable of deciding things for themselves.

In other words, you have taken away their MAJOR strength of self-confidence.

Behind their confused behaviour is an intelligent, capable person with a lifetime of experience and memories, which can be re-stimulated with skilled attention.

If you reflect on whether YOU are controlling and find that you are, ask yourself; "Am I controlling to meet my OWN needs?"

Try to write a note for yourself.

Who does my controlling help most? Me?

_____

_____

_____

_____

_____

_____

_____

_____

_____

_____

Asking questions

There can be few habits more dominating in the world! It is second nature to the human race.

To a so-called normal person, being questioned, within reason, is perfectly acceptable.

"How are you today dear?"

"Would you like a cup of tea?'"

"Have you taken your pills?"

"What would you like for dinner?"

"Would you like to go for a walk?"

"What would you like to wear today?"

"Have you washed today dear?'"

To the person doubting their sanity, it is TORTURE.

It will PROVOKE rage, which will either exploded in your face or be turned inwards to cause stubborn resistance and a refusal to listen or co-operate.

Over the next few days, count the number of times you ask questions and the frequency.

Length of time in the presence of ....
.... *(cared-for person)*

Number of questions asked ....

Frequency ....

What reactions did I get? Please continue with this exercise until you have learned how to phrase questions in a way, which do not cause negative reactions.

<u>YOUR QUESTIONING EXERCISE</u>

In order to comprehend the effect questioning may have on the cared-for person, please reflect on your OWN past examination experiences. Do you remember how you felt when the exam question left you totally confused? How you really dreaded facing questions! Panic set in!

For this exercise please spend one day listening to the questions around you and count.

THIS IS HOW MANY:

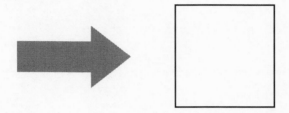

Please refrain from asking questions with your cared-for person. They have the same effect you felt when you panicked at your exams. Learn the trick of implying: "I think I am going to make myself a cup of tea."

Have I reduced the number of questions I am throwing at (name the person)?

_____

_____

_____

_____

_____

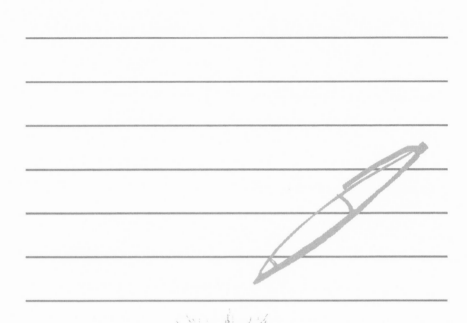

Irritating

In the 'real world', irritating someone, or being irritated, is frequently little more than teasing and in the family it is acknowledged as something we do to each other. On the other hand, it can be a personality feature about which we have very little awareness.

In dementia world, it becomes a borderline feature which can be expressed with laughter, as a funny moment or a thoughtless act towards someone whose ability to think quickly and comprehend meaning, has deserted them.

In this exercise please make discreet enquiries amongst your CLOSE friends and relatives and ask them:

"What is it about ME that irritates YOU the most?"

Findings here please: (the chances of you learning from this depend upon your new, calm and relaxed manner!)

....

....

....

....

....

YOUR IRRITATION EXERCISE

This is a mannerism, which most of us react to either by escaping from the irritant or demanding that it goes away. However, the irritating person frequently doesn't know about it. Even when they are told, they may cease for a while, but gradually return to their irritating mannerisms.

In normal everyday relations we all get used to these little things and tend to ignore them, or just brush them off as "one of HIS things!"

The questions for us working through these exercises are; "Am I irritating, but not aware of it and how does it affect the person for whom I care, experiencing dementia?"

As this is the last exercise, it calls for sincere self-discovery which also requires courage.

You have to approach your friends very skillfully and without them feeling confronted by you, find out if you ARE irritating, and if so, in what way.

Try to write a few notes about your discovery.

Do people find me irritating? Can I change?

Becoming a good conductor

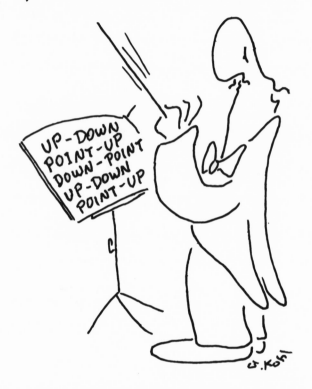

I have two very important relevant memories about conducting.

There was a four year period in my teens, when I attended orchestra practice once per week, playing my clarinet under the same conductor. We were always very pleased with ourselves, except on the occasions when visiting, professional conductors stood in. The difference was truly amazing! We all used to end the evening by saying; *"Why don't we play like that when Bob (our regular conductor) conducts?"*

The second conductor revelation came through my own training as a group analyst. Group analysis is where a group of eight people experiencing emotional problems, learn how to overcome them though their interactions with each other. Our group conductor, the accepted term for a group analytic professional, conducted us every week and our 'performance' gradually acquired a level where I knew I was learning the skills of a group conductor.

In the same way as in my teens experience, the visiting professional conductor supervised me for my own groups. He was the profoundly wise and experienced founder of the Group Analytic movement in London.*

* *Dr. S.H. Foulkes*

The difference was truly amazing! I was consistently astonished by the insights I developed into the behaviour and the interactions of my groups. Why couldn't I perform with the same expertise in my training group?

The two conductors in my life had been profoundly skilled through doing and learning what has to be done to create the harmonious results they had learned to achieve.

Everyone learns by DOING things.

Unless you have acquired skills from doing the exercises so far and can now get quickly into a happy state, there is NO point going any further!

Remember, this is a Be-It-Yourself workbook. You are NOT DOING anything to anybody but yourself.

In order to create that amazingly harmonious atmosphere for the whole orchestra, great conductors need to KNOW certain things before they take to the rostrum.

Like what the best version of the music they are conducting SOUNDS like, from having heard it in the past.

Also like what each instrument SHOULD be playing, its specific sounds and its melodic contribution to the whole.

They learn to encourage every single musician to play with inspiration and experience the joy and elation of being immersed in a harmonious atmosphere.

We have looked at the twelve habits, beliefs and mannerisms lurking around a normal relationship which can cause havoc in dementia world.

I sincerely hope that you have introduced more well-being in the home and that dementia world is beginning to feel *less* stressful.

Following the next set of exercises will add to your expertise and turn you into a brilliant conductor of interpersonal behaviour!

Composing the symphony

We now know that any ONE of the hand grenades below can have an explosive effect on interpersonal relations even with so-called *normal* people.

Opinionating

Interrupting

Provoking Contrdicting

Expecting gratitude

Talking Loudly

Undermining

Pessimism

Ignoring Need to control

Questioning

Irritating

Hopefully we have gained expertise and can now conduct our relations with skilled awareness. But it doesn't mean that all will now be peace and goodwill!

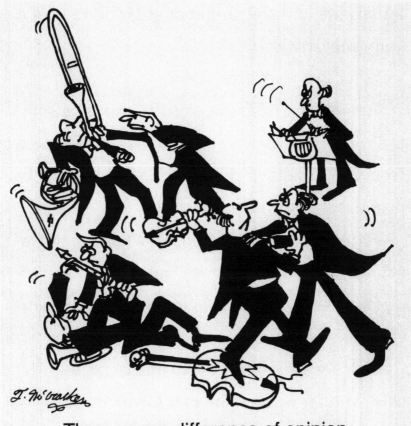

There was a difference of opinion
on how to play the second movement.

The one thing a great conductor will NOT do, is choose a composition which would prove to be completely impossible for him to conduct!

Imagine that *you* are going to conduct an orchestra. There are feelings you must have if you want to bring the very best out of the musicians and the audience is going to give a standing ovation.

What are your priorities?

You, on the rostrum, your baton is raised, tap it on the music stand and begin to conduct from the music score in front of you which is profoundly familiar to you.

You know that you KNOW what the score sounds like when it is well-conducted. You also know what your home is like when YOU sense a state of well-being.

Now I want you to take time to pause, close your eyes, and on as many occasions you can, create a scene which is equivalent to you listening to your favourite calming music.

Refresh the memories, people, places, activities, objects which instinctively change your EXISTING feelings.

The following exercises will construct a 'symphony of notes' which when played within the interpersonal world of your daily living, transform the discordant noises of an untutored 'band' to an harmonious 'ensemble'!

The first exercise is FOR YOU to go through what follows and by so doing, compose your own symphony. *(Do not forget, this is a BE-IT-YOURSELF book!)*

The vital and critical reason for this is that you are a UNIQUE person with UNIQUE feelings which are associated with YOUR unique lifelong experiences.

Until YOU have composed your own symphony and learned how to enjoy it, you will not know HOW to conduct the symphony which is laying in the lifelong well-being experiences of ANYONE ELSE.

If you are living with, and caring for, a person experiencing some form of dementia, the use of these UNIQUE, instinctive promoters of well-being are the difference between the black hole of despondency and daily moments of good cheer and happy interpersonal relations.

There is a state of mind, in addition to the calm state you will have by now been able to achieve, which is of EQUAL importance and that is in your conviction about the totally unique life experiences of the person you care for with dementia.

Their *UNIQUENESS* is the *treasure chest which belongs only to the person with dementia. Carers who know how to detect and use the treasures, will most definitely have found the path to well-being.*

(Those who invent are likely to come up against fierce resistance after the initial and 'apparent' success).

Distinguished interaction

We know the standard of interaction between people which can be described as "normal" contains our twelve hand grenades.

During a trip to different locations in India and Australia, it struck me very forcibly that these grenade interactions were totally acceptable in many care settings.

I then realised that UNLESS the carers could distinguish between their normal grenade interactions and sensitive thoughtful interactions, they could not make any improvements in the quality of life for their cared-for people.

We are all like fish in a fishbowl who cannot know they are in water. Instead of water, we are *swimming* in a medium of linguistic interactions which can cause us to be very harmful towards each other without knowing we are doing it.

We CANNOT know what effect interactive habits we use naturally are having on those of us whose brains are diseased, *unless* we get out of the fishbowl, and by observing our fellow fish, distinguish their grenade behaviour!

Seeing it objectively, and the effects it is causing, will eventually build up distinguished responses instead of explosions.

When we are outside looking in at our *fellow fish* inside the bowl, creating explosive interactions, we CAN know what to do differently. Their behaviour is blatantly obvious and the effect they are causing is equally, blatantly obvious.

But ONLY from the outside looking in!

Let us take our twelve grenades and look at our fellow fish in the bowl.

OPINIONATING

"Isn't s/he crude! Fancy imposing their opinion

on that poor person, who can hardly sustain a single opinion about anything. Why don't they let them express their own opinions and AGREE with them, instead of trying to impose their own opinions?"

INTERRUPTING

"Can you tell them NOT to keep interrupting? The poor man can't even finish a sentence *without* being interrupted! They are making it ten times worse by not letting him finish his sentences."

Give him time and space to express his opinion – *and agree with him!*

PROVOCATION

" Isn't it amazing that they CAN'T see what is provoking him? They only have to see his expression when they take him past that photo of his pet dog which died years ago."

CONTRADICTION

"He is really struggling to make sense of what is

going on around him, and that carer will NOT stop contradicting everything he says!

Can't they see he is on thin ice with his own state of mind? He doesn't need people to go on contradicting him."

EXPECTING GRATITUDE

Oh no! Surely they have recognised he has gone passed knowing what they are doing for him. Why are they still asking for his approval?
"Did you like that George?" *LIKE WHAT?*

The carer should be expressing her gratitude to him.

"George, you are wonderful, it is so nice being with you."

TALKING LOUDLY

Does a distinguished person EVER talk loudly? When the art of distinguished interaction is mastered, talking loudly, unless the person has difficulty hearing, is an insult to anyone.

UNDERMINING

From outside the fishbowl we see a person whose confidence is being shattered daily to such an extent, that they are increasingly asking questions such as, "Where am I?"

Telling them they know that already or surely you know George etc. adds to the demolition of their self-confidence. *Another nail in their coffin!*

PESSIMISM

The most pervasive, contagious behaviour trait in so-called civilized society.

Bus queues, old people's homes' day-rooms, staff rooms, it is everywhere.

From the outside, what do *YOU* do? Join it, ignore it, positively counteract it?

IGNORING

How could anyone do this if they are really distinguishing the acute need for attention and understanding in the cared-for person?

CONTROLLING

"Come on Dad, I will sign that for you."

"Let me find you a shirt to put on darling."

"I have been signing and putting on my bl....dy
shirts ALL my life!!"

ASKING QUESTIONS.

"Here I am with this bl....dy dementia creeping
in and I am having huge difficulty making sense
of everything, and this bl....dy person won't stop
asking me questions! Do I want this, do I want
that, have I shaved? Have I taken my pills?
Will they EVER stop?"

Don't confuse even more!

IRRITATING

"Oh no" not her again!

We, from the outside, see that the carer has at
least three acutely irritating mannerisms. *Has
anyone told her?*

We can see that Joyce ALWAYS averts her
attention from the photo of her son. Why?

The GP always walks in wearing a stethoscope..!

THE DISTINGUISHED INTERACTION IMPERATIVE

Unless we keep the twelve hand grenades firmly in our memory and diffuse them, the minute we see them being thrown, we are just as guilty as our colleagues in the 'fishbowl.'

There is ever increasing evidence that exercising distinguished interaction, transforms the well-being of EVERYONE, either using it or experiencing it with an intelligent, aware person.

"My husband is beginning to hear me. The other day he asked if I was alright!"

"Dad, actually asked for my opinion!"

"My Mum started to tell me things she had never mentioned to me before."

"He hadn't spoken to any of us for weeks and all of a sudden, asked me who I was !"

The benefits extend beyond the interactions.

Inspiring re-inspiration

There is a profound difference between a caring manner which calls upon known skills and techniques and tuning into the inspirational moments of your cared-for person.

As we mentioned, *you* have to rediscover *your own* moments of inspiration and carry the feelings they arouse in *you* into the presence of your cared-for person.

The profound difference arises from a quality which we ALL possess but which remains in the *"twilight zone"* of our toolbox!

Common sense people tend to dismiss it as ridiculous nonsense, dementia sense people who experience it every day, would call it *uncanny*.

We can ALL sense something we might call an intuitive awareness and it is common to hear people saying "I *knew* that would happen!"

Or, "You've taken the words right out of my mouth!"

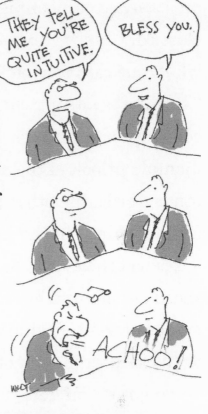

This type of contact between people has been described as synchronicity and there are books full of the history and frequency of it. Most of us, *know* about but have dismissed it as a *weird* happening.

I am ADVOCATING it for this age of behaviour, associated with the new era of prolonged life symptoms. Until recently, they were considered as old-age problems. They are ***not*** old-age problems, they ***are*** new, age problems.

As soon as we notice that certain types of event "like" to cluster together at certain times, we begin to understand the attitude of the Chinese, whose theories of medicine are based on a *science* of meaningful coincidences. The classical Chinese texts did not ask what causes what, but rather what *likes* to occur with what. This represents a tremendous problem for our conventional thinkers, because it requires the mental outlook of the *participant observer.* In other words, the other person and *you* generate a "happening" in the same way as Einstein described the events happening on the time/space continuum.

The absolutely vital essence of truly tuning in to the inspirational moments of your cared-for person, rests on how you have to been able to *transmit your own inspirational feelings.*

When you begin to share any of your own moments of inspiration, it will, sooner or later, mostly to your own great surprise, re-stimulate an *inspirational feeling* in your cared-for person. This can happen around any of the four 'p's which *you* take with you to start the 'meeting'.

Over time, you will have detected some clues

about the inspirational people, places, pastimes and possessions which have shown themselves in your cared-for person.

E.g. "I met Frank Smith in the newspaper shop this morning."

(Remember how you feel about a person in YOUR moments of inspiration and that you know the cared-for person has Frank Smith in their experience).

"Oh! Did you? How is he?"

(The inspired moment has been re-inspired and usually a whole scenario around Frank Smith and what they did together etc., will arise).

You love gardening; "I am having great difficulty with my ...."

(You know gardening is an inspirational pastime. Give yourself time, RELAX and synchronicity strikes again)!

Your cared-for person will probably smile and even start telling you how much trouble they used to have with.....

There are people who would dismiss this style of caring on the grounds that advanced dementia appears to make a person incapable of speaking and using intuition is a waste of time. They tend to be *common sense* people!

On the contrary, it is my experience that this sensitive transmission of *personal inspirational experience* is more effective with apparently closed down people.

When you carry in a sense of "I would *love* to see how we start," it frequently re-stimulates, even without having any knowledge of the person's inspirational moments.

Complete the following exercise, *trust your intuition,* combine your inspirational moments with the distinguished interaction of grenade-free meetings *...and see transitions!*

People, pastimes, possessions and places

It is thought by students of Vivaldi that much of the inspiration for his violin concertos, Four Seasons, came from his observations of the location in which he spent three years near Mantua, Italy.

What makes this music *revolutionary* is his detailed observations of minor, almost insignificant occurrences and their inclusion into the composition.

If we, in turn, make the same detailed observations of our four most incident filled life occurrences, however trivial they may seem to anyone else, TO YOU they have become your concerto. They, as Vivaldi observed, CONSTITUTE the concerto. *(If the Four Seasons Concerto is not familiar to you, you should give yourself the pleasure of hearing it).*

Please note YOU are opening experiences with feelings, which instantaneously evoke instinctive responses of well-being.

There is a discipline to this exercise. As I mentioned earlier in the calming exercise, you have to let your mind wander through your childhood, just let it wander!

Like fishing, you will catch old boots or bike frames occasionally which you discard with disgust! Then, all of a sudden, you burst into spontaneous laughter because you *catch* a very beautiful experience. It could be funny, romantic, awe-inspiring, happy, crying or proud but it is unique to YOU and it is spontaneous.

Keep doing this every day. DO NOT hang on to the negative stuff you might hook. Throw it away! You MUST work hard NOT TO cling on to negative experiences.

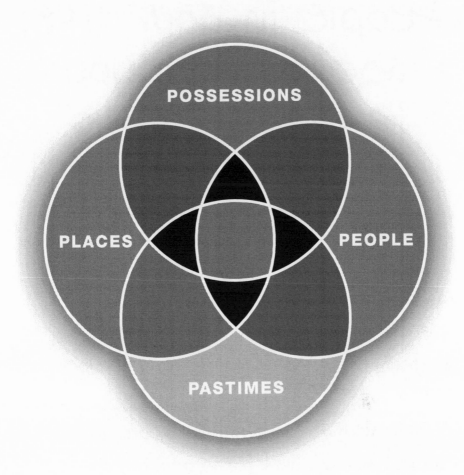

These are the worlds
where moments you treasure
combine and constitute the
'symphony' of YOUR life.

People in your life about whom you have registered pleasant experiences

Again, YOU are going to BE and try to identify your own people experiences, BEFORE trying to reveal those which your cared-for person may reveal.

Start with earliest family members; uncles, aunts, schoolteachers, playground friends, shopkeepers, doctors, vicars, next-door-neighbours, etc.

Really get INTO this exercise yourself because you will be truly astonished when you look at the list of names AND the associated feelings attached to them!

This exercise will rekindle many feelings and people you may have thought that you had forgotten. Please note that we are looking ONLY for those which bring a smile and clear memories of the good times your have experienced.

You will have to write them down and ensure only the BEST are recorded. These are three of my many promoters of well-being!

My teacher. We used to tease our maths teacher because we knew he would throw chalk at us. We learned to duck!

My friend Chloe NEVER paid attention but she ALWAYS knew the answer when Mrs Dixon surprised her. We always laughed.

Uncle George was hilarious. I laughed everytime he visited us. He used to stand behind a door and talk like Mr Punch.

Great fun!

Who caused me to laugh?

Pastimes which always cause you to feel good

On walks, experiencing learning, sports, passing exams, driving test, games you played. Journeys.

Again it is vital that YOU be there and experience those feelings.

Swimming, riding, learning, tasting, seeing, meeting, celebrating, being praised, falling in love . . .

These occasions will evoke spontaneous smiles, laughter and well-being reactions.

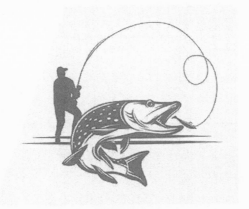

What pastimes have always made me feel good?

Possessions with which you have some special familiarity

This is a very special exercise because there is every possibility that objects with special attachments will go back a very long way and will evoke whole scenarios of memories and feelings.

Its use is also extremely valuable to restore well-being and bring our cared-for person into a higher state of well-being.

Please go back into your own childhood, starting with the first object you recall.
e.g. exercise book, toy soldier, banana, doll, pet, Easter egg, painting set, toy microscope, scooter, bike, ball, fishing rod, apple, ring, magazine, etc.

The KEY here is that these objects will strike a chord as forcibly as the key a conductor asks the orchestra to play in order to bring it into harmony. *The effect is magic!*

What possessions have always made me laugh?

Places where you have experienced happy feelings from childhood onwards

The seaside.

The circus.

The zoo.

A campsite.

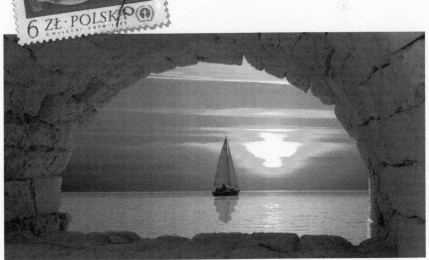

What places have made me laugh?

In BIG letters, please transfer the ESSENTIAL laughter-inducing highlights you have written on the previous four 'Ps'. They are THE one's which never fail to make you laugh or at least smile.

This list, and more as you add more, will be your masterpiece to immediately inspire you and recharge your energy. Don't forget! They have to induce NATURAL instantaneous responses.

_____

_____

_____

_____

_____

_____

_____

_____

_____

"What inspires you? Store
it in a place in your heart
and use it for energy"

Sir Richard Branson.
Twitter, 7 June 2012

Encore

I have been very privileged to attend hundreds of *performances* of family members and live-in carers conducting their day-to-day caring and using their unique understanding of the cared-for person.

Each one was like observing different orchestras playing the same concerto. The conductors bring their own interpretation to the piece.

There are three consistent conducting skills which always seem to bring out the best performance. It is the same reason why great conductors always have a huge following conducting any great orchestra. They KNOW the music and composers intimately!

The same principle applies to our loved one. At EVERY performance there is:

1. The projection of a calm, understanding

presence. The calmness is expressed through a gentle voice and smooth physical movement.

2. Waiting for the cared-for person to lead the way.

3. Very sharp attention and response to gestures or expressions, which bring well-being emotions into the moment.

One final use of our conducting metaphor

Leaving the room of someone experiencing dementia has to be conducted with the skill based on your knowledge of THEIR knowledge of YOU.

It has been my experience on hundreds of occasions to see the crushing effect departing carers or relatives have caused.

Remember, we are leaving someone who might be in a very fragile, confused and anxious condition where their reality could explode.

Your presence will have raised their sense of well-being higher than usual.

How do they feel when the
conductor leaves?
If the conductor doesn't re-assure them?
If they sense they may never
see the conductor again?

Don't forget, they have experienced a *great sense of well being!*

Our cared-for person NEEDS to know that you are leaving to do something they know you always do!

E.g. they know you always pop out to do some shopping....and come back.

They always know you have a class to teach... and always come back.

DO NOT leave them with MORE confusion.

Whatever your departing words are, they tune precisely into what they KNOW you do.

How do you conduct yourself now – after the exercises?

A second shot at the survey will enable you to compare your results now, with your initial results on page 18 and see if they have changed.

There has been some delightful feedback from many people who have completed it the second time, especially family members who are caring for someone experiencing dementia. Reports such as *"he is telling us things about his life which we had never heard before and about places we never knew he had visited"*.

There is no doubt that when they spend enough time consciously changing their interactions with the cared-for person, they also begin to change their interactions with each other.

ON A SCALE OF 1-10, HOW FREQUENTLY DO I NOW . . .

	1	2	3	4	5	6	7	8	9	10
Opinionate:	☐	☐	☐	☐	☐	☐	☐	☐	☐	☐
Interrupt:	☐	☐	☐	☐	☐	☐	☐	☐	☐	☐
Provoke:	☐	☐	☐	☐	☐	☐	☐	☐	☐	☐
Contradict:	☐	☐	☐	☐	☐	☐	☐	☐	☐	☐
Expect Gratitude:	☐	☐	☐	☐	☐	☐	☐	☐	☐	☐
Talk Loudly:	☐	☐	☐	☐	☐	☐	☐	☐	☐	☐
Undermine:	☐	☐	☐	☐	☐	☐	☐	☐	☐	☐
Act Pessimistic:	☐	☐	☐	☐	☐	☐	☐	☐	☐	☐
Ignore:	☐	☐	☐	☐	☐	☐	☐	☐	☐	☐
Control:	☐	☐	☐	☐	☐	☐	☐	☐	☐	☐
Ask Questions:	☐	☐	☐	☐	☐	☐	☐	☐	☐	☐
Irritate:	☐	☐	☐	☐	☐	☐	☐	☐	☐	☐

A client phoned to tell me, that noticing how much he was interrupting and opinionating with his wife and children he had suddenly realized, having stopped, that he was now having lengthy, intelligent conversations and his wife had become much more interesting!

The VITAL point here is that everything we

do for our loved one comes from our deep need to do the best we can.

When our COMMON SENSE acquires a thoughtful, considered dementia sense, our natural, everyday language, instead of causing added confusion and intense emotions, can transform ALL relationships - not just those we have with our cared-for person.

"Any intelligent fool can make things bigger and more complex.
It takes a touch of genius and a lot of courage to move in the opposite direction"

Albert Einstein

Conclusions

There can be nothing worse in everyday life than living in circumstances which seem impossible to understand, or from which you cannot escape.

The three aspects of care I am advocating, understand the effects of linguistic interactions which I describe as *'hand grenades'*. Developing *distinguished interaction* as a result of our awareness and *inspiring re-inspiration,* hopefully add to the current brilliant practices in dementia care.

Over the many years of hearing the words 'nightmare' or 'black hole' being expressed by exhausted wives, husbands, sons and daughters, I found through long hours of calming MY mind that there are routes out of the nightmare.

These pages are in no way the definitive route map but I know that YOU have to practice calming to become an expert in dementia world.

Any action which does not involve YOU being in the cared-for person's state of mind on FREQUENT occasions is likely to create problems, rather than smooth the situation.

It is no good staying detached! Living the reality is totally different from part-time caring.

It will hurt like hell until you have learned dementia world language and behaviour. When you have, you find that you transcend the nightmare and relate to people with a calm confidence you may never have imagined yourself having.

You REGAIN a self which can look back at your common sense world and smile at the *games* being played!

The twelve hand grenades are NORMAL everyday interactions to us but NOT to those experiencing dementia.

The moments of profound pleasure are UNIQUE to the person for whom you are caring.

Hopefully this simple book will have done a good job and you now feel more optimistic and enlightened.

Kindest regards

Appendix

Relaxation is an art, a state of mind, something that seems to elude us when we need it and which we need to practice in these busy and pressured times.

There are many different types and methods of relaxation and meditation. I would urge the reader to explore the different types and adapt them to find strategies that work for them, remembering that often one strategy will not work all the time, so several may be used in conjunction with each other.

A simple method to use is to carry a small, smooth pebble in your pocket so that each time you place your hand into your pocket you feel the coolness and smoothness of the pebble which may make you stop for a moment and mindfully, just enjoy the sensation, focus on a word, or happy moments you have held in your memory. For those few seconds, as you roll the pebble around in your palm, you may be transported from the crowded train, the meeting or the person shouting demands at you. Happy thoughts allow you to re-join the present with a smile or a deep breath and carry on.

That leads to another method of relaxation and quieting the mind; breathing. It is something we take for granted and goes unnoticed, however, as we become more tense or anxious our breathing becomes more shallow and rapid. To slow the breathing down can help us to feel calmer. Focusing on our breathing for just a couple of minutes helps us leave the anxious, negative thoughts behind.

For a deeper spell of relaxation, make yourself comfortable sitting in a chair or lying on the bed or floor. Snuggle down and settle your body so that it feels limp, then carry on with the following ideas.

Begin by letting your breath out and then

breathe in as far as you want. Wait for just a moment, then breathe out slowly relaxing into the chair, bed or floor, as you do so. Do this once more, very slowly and, as you breathe out, feel the tension draining away. Now go back to your ordinary breathing. Keep it even, calm, easy, then forget about it.

Lindsey Skelt Dip. C.O.T.

www.shires-therapy.co.uk

Some readers may find that Alison Bourne's methods of relaxation and meditation detailed in her comprehensive work; *Colour Breathing* are ideal for them.

For details visit: *www.colourbreathing.com*

Printed in Great Britain
by Amazon.co.uk, Ltd.,
Marston Gate.